KATHRYN MARSDEN

D1578585

Hotline to Health

PAN BOOKS

First published 1998 by Pan Books
an imprint of Macmillan Publishers Ltd
25 Eccleston Place, London SW1W 9NF
and Basingstoke

Associated companies throughout the world

ISBN 0 330 35369 1

A CIP catalogue record for this book is available from
the British Library.

Typeset by SX Composing DTP, Rayleigh, Essex
Printed and bound in Great Britain by
Mackays of Chatham plc, Chatham, Kent

This edition was specially produced for *Zest* magazine by arrangement
with Pan Books. The full and unabridged edition is available at all good
bookshops, or by using the order form at the back of this book.

ADVICE TO THE READER
Before following any medical or dietary advice contained in this book, it is
recommended that you consult your doctor if you suffer from any health
problems or special conditions or are in any doubt as to its suitability.

I'm delighted to bring *Zest* readers this exclusive edition of Kathryn Marsden's new book, *Hotline to Health*. It offers constructive help for common health problems such as allergies, candida and PMS.

The author of the bestselling *Food Combining Diet, Food Combining in 30 Days* and *Super Skin*, Kathryn has years of experience in the field of nutritional health. *Hotline to Health* is packed with anecdotes, tips, advice and self-help suggestions that Kathryn has gleaned from her work, and I'm sure you'll find it both enjoyable and useful.

Eve Cameron
Editor
Zest magazine

Contents

୬

Healthy Woman

⁓

Pre-Menstrual Tension Syndrome

PMTS is a hormonally related condition of a cyclical nature characterized by a long list of extremely unpleasant symptoms. It's been estimated that there could be 300 or more symptoms associated with PMTS (which can occur several days before, just before and even during a period) although, apparently, it's unlikely anyone would suffer with all of them at once! I can't actually think of that many, so thank goodness for something. They can include:

Abdominal bloating
Agoraphobia
Anxiety
Bad hair days
Breast tenderness
Cramps
Cravings
Crying
Poor concentration
Poor coordination
Depression

Emotional disturbance
Fluid retention
Forgetfulness
Need for frequent meals
Headaches
Irrational hostility
Irritable bowel
Irritable behaviour
Lack of energy
Lethargy
Migraine
Mood swings
Murderous thoughts
Palpitations
Panic attacks
Sleep problems
Skin flare-ups
Excessive thirst
Excessive sweating
Shivering
Acute stress
Twisted tights!
Nothing fits!
Outbursts of temper
and
Weight gain
often accompanied by the strong desire to tear out
your hair and throw your complete wardrobe into
the street

So what's the cause?

Menstrual, pre-menstrual and menopausal disorders are almost certainly, to use a useful medical term, multifactorial; meaning that there are probably several factors involved. There may, indeed, be a psychological aspect but, after all the research that has been carried out, it seems fairly likely that hormones are the major player in this scenario!

Ah, you guessed.

All in the mind . . . Again?

A group of psychiatrists in the US have, however, attempted recently to turn familiar old pre-menstrual tension into a certifiable mental illness called PMDD ('pre-menstrual dysphoric disorder'), previously known as 'late luteal phase dysphoric disorder'.

Rolls off the tongue nice and easily, don't you think?

A storm of protest ensued from a variety of learned (female) quarters that the evidence for this diagnosis was lousy. PMDD, if it exists at all, describes only a tiny percentage of the female population. The psychiatrists (I am told that they are all men!) wriggled and coughed and climbed down from their perch but couldn't really see what all the fuss was about. No need for women to get on their high horses, their spokesman replied pithily.

And the result of all this aggro?

The new 'category' was swiftly delisted and relisted as requiring 'further study'. Well, thanks a lot, guys!

Unfair assessments

Why label pre-menstrual tension a mental illness at all? There are plenty of physical illnesses which cause changes in mood and behaviour. When we are depressed by a heavy dose of the flu, we don't call it chronic influenza dysphoric depressive disorder; well, do we?

Real physical reasons

Now fairly well known, I think, but included here for those who aren't aware of his work: Dr Guy Abraham, former Professor of Obstetrics and Gynaecology at the University of California Los Angeles, has carried out a number of studies into pre-menstrual problems and come up with guidelines suggesting that symptoms can be subdivided into four main groups. Not definitive, of course, but useful in illustrating the difficulties faced both by doctors and sufferers in trying to diagnose the condition. The notes are intended only as a guide; sufferers can be affected by symptoms from one or all groups.

If you suffer with PMTS-A, you are likely to experience:

ANXIETY
Disturbed sleep
Irritability
Mood swings
Nervous tension
Panic attacks

PMTS-A has been linked to increased levels of oestrogen and reduced levels of progesterone. Too much sugar and dairy products may aggravate symptoms even more. It's good to include more foods rich in B vitamins if this is your kind of PMT. How about avocado, dried fruits, brown rice, oats, all kinds of vegetables and salads, oily fish, yoghurt, free-range eggs and pulses?

PMTS-B manifests symptoms such as:

BLOATING
Fluid retention
Distended abdomen
Breast pain/tenderness
Swollen ankles
Weight gain
Irritable bladder
Irritable bowel
Constipation

PMTS-B is sometimes listed as PMTS-H (meaning *Hyperhydration*). This 'watery' kind of hormonal imbalance may benefit from extra Vitamins E, B complex and the mineral chromium. Up your intake of asparagus, beetroot, cheese, chicken, eggs, seafood, nuts, seeds, vegetables, cold-pressed oils, wholegrains, soya beans and greens. Avoid coffee, tea, cola, chocolate, cigarette smoke and salt.

The third group, PMTS-C, stands for:

CRAVINGS
Dizziness
Fainting spells
Headaches
Hunger
Migraine
Palpitations
Sudden fatigue

**Blood sugar disturbance is a key factor in PMTS-C. Foods
rich in minerals magnesium (fresh and dried fruits,
brown rice, bananas, fish, root ginger, lemons, pasta and
pulses) and chromium (above) can be helpful. So, too, can
essential fatty acids such as those found in cold-pressed
oils, oily fish, seeds, nuts and in supplements made from
borage oil and evening primrose oil. In this type of PMT,
there may sometimes be an intolerance to certain types
of foods so improving the digestion and removing common allergens are both useful steps to take.**

PMTS-D, the fourth group, indicates:

DEPRESSION
Crying
Confusion
Poor co-ordination
Insomnia
Forgetfulness
Loss of perspective

Progesterone levels may be higher than normal in PMTS-D. Heavy metal toxicity – especially lead – has been discovered by some researchers. Foods rich in B vitamins, calcium, magnesium and selenium are recommended. Go for wholegrains, all kinds of fish, green and root vegetables, sunflower and pumpkin seeds, almonds, Brazils, onions, tomatoes and garlic.

Menstrual Mayhem

For some lucky souls, menstruation happens lightly and conveniently for two to four days in a (set-your-watch-by-it) 28-day rotation. For many others, the 'monthly cycle' is a distant dream. Periods can be irregular, infrequent, too frequent, too heavy, painful or non-existent. However, just because your period lasts for seven days and the woman at the next desk is over and done with in three – or you have a 26-day cycle when someone else can count five or six weeks – doesn't mean your cycle is abnormal. Normal is what is normal for you when you are feeling fit and well.

MAKING SENSE OF THE TERMINOLOGY:

Amenorrhoea means lack of periods

Dysmenorrhoea means painful periods

Menorrhagia means heavy periods

Metrorrhagia is bleeding between periods

Mittelschmerz translates as 'middle pain' and indicates ovulation pain

Oligomenorrhoea is the medical term for sporadic, infrequent periods

Polymenorrhoea means abnormally frequent periods

Are your periods a pain?

If there have been any sudden or unusual changes in the characteristics, intensity or frequency of your periods or you feel unwell during menstruation when you usually feel fine, then do see your doctor without delay.

Fibroids, ovarian cysts, endometriosis, adenomyosis (endometriosis in the muscle wall of the womb), pelvic adhesions or the potentially more hazardous pelvic inflammatory disease can all cause painful menstruation.

Periods may be considered abnormal if pain has been lasting longer than usual, is more intense, occurs in a different place, occurs at times other than your period, is accompanied by other symptoms or is not improved by normal pain medication at normal doses.

Heavy periods

If your flow is heavy every time, the blood loss could lead to borderline anaemia without realizing there is a problem. However, as I have cautioned so many times in the past, don't take iron supplements without first going to your GP for a test. Excess iron can be as dangerous as a deficiency; in other words, don't take it if you don't need it.

Make sure your diet has plenty of foods which contain iron (naturally occurring, not artificially 'fortified'), such as dark green vegetables and salad foods, dried fruit, oats, pulses and seafood. Raw beetroot is a valuable source and makes an excellent blood tonic. For those who don't like the taste, capsules of beetroot extract are available from Biocare.

Testing thyroid

I have seen a number of cases where those with painful or heavy periods, suddenly scant periods, severe PMTS, infertility or unresolved menopausal difficulties were found to have either an overactive or underactive thyroid. Many PMTS symptoms show a striking similarity to those of thyroid imbalance. So if you're experiencing any unsolved health problems (difficulties maintaining a balanced weight, palpitations, persistent tiredness, irritable bowel, depression or restlessness, for example), do talk to your doctor who may suggest some tests.

Candida connection

Candidiasis and heavy periods sometimes go together, too. But avoid strict anti-candida diets which can disturb the cycle, causing bleeding between periods or stopping them altogether.

Periods slowed or stopped?

If you have always had light or infrequent periods and

you feel generally well, then there should be no cause for concern. However, if your periods have recently become infrequent or have ceased completely, ask yourself what lifestyle changes you have made over the past few months. For example, have you been under extra stress, been following one or more low-calorie diets or overdoing the exercise? All these factors can lead to amenorrhoea or oligomenorrhoea.

It has been publicized only relatively recently that athletes and other sports enthusiasts can suffer with 'runner's amenorrhoea' where periods cease altogether. Excessive exercise puts additional stress on the body and can deplete the system of several vital nutrients, particularly iron and Vitamin C.

Help is at hand

Providing that there is no underlying medical problem, it has been my experience that following the nutritional and other hints which begin on page 46 will usually return difficult or absent periods to normal within four to six months for most women.

Did you know that . . .
The first documented operation to remove an ovarian cyst was performed in 1809 in Danville, Kentucky, USA, by Dr Ephraim McDowell. There being no anaesthetic available in those days, the patient sustained herself by singing hymns. She survived.

Endometriosis

Endometriosis happens when pieces of stray tissue from the lining of the womb (the endometrium) set up in other sites such as the bladder, fallopian tubes, intestines or ovaries.

In response to normal hormonal changes, the lining of the uterus grows, bleeds and sheds. Unfortunately, the tissue which 'got away' also grows and bleeds, too – but is trapped and unable to shed. As a result there is congestion, scarring, adhesions of the pelvic organs (they stick together) and often very severe pain. If left untreated, endometriosis can also lead to infertility.

As far as causes are concerned, fingers have been pointed at oestrogen excess, progesterone deficiency, immune-system suppression, and toxic overload from drug medications or environmental pollutants.

Pre-conceptual connection

Another theory is that endometriosis begins in the unborn child. Endometrial cells laid down before birth may end up in the wrong place but no one knows until they make their presence felt when activated at puberty.

Toxic interference

The foetus can also be affected by toxins from medicines or pollution. For example:

Dioxins

Dioxins, dangerous chemicals produced from chlorine waste products, are a prime suspect. When these airborne contaminants fall on to grass and crops, they then find their way into the human food chain. In one particular study, the incidence of endometriosis was connected directly to dioxin exposure. The stronger the dose of dioxin, the worse the endometriosis!

Kathryn Marsden's new book *The Food Combining 2-Day Detox* contains additional information on dioxins and the best way to protect the body from chemical overload.

Operations

Abdominal surgery can sometimes trigger the travel of endometrial tissue into other areas of the body – worth adding to your list of possibles if your problems have occurred since an operation for a related or unrelated condition.

The period connection

There is some evidence that the number of periods a woman has may determine whether or not she risks endometriosis. It is estimated that in hunter–gatherer times women probably had only thirty or so menstrual periods and a maximum of six children. Fast forward to the reign of Queen Victoria and we find females producing anything up to eighteen children and experiencing a hundred periods. In our time, most women have 450 or more menstrual cycles but on average only two children. So the ratio of periods to babies born has altered radically in only a few thousand years from 1:5 to 1:225. Doctors are interested in how these changes in fertility and hormone production may influence endometriosis.

Other possibilities

Links have also been suggested between endometriosis and sexual abuse, relationship difficulties, feelings of inadequacy, excessive stress, candidiasis or allergies.

Hormone drugs

If you suffer or have suffered from the condition, be aware that both HRT and the Pill could trigger or reactivate endometriosis. I have interviewed a number of practitioners who are concerned about the long-term effects of hormone drugs. Australian naturopath Ross Trattler, in his book *Better Health Through Natural Healing*, states: 'Probably the most effective way to upset the entire hormonal system is to take the birth control pill.'

Runs in families

And the condition may run in families, so, if possible, try to find out what symptoms your mother or grandmother experienced.

What to look for

If you have ongoing, heavy or painful periods that don't respond to treatment, a bowel or bladder which becomes 'irritable' just before or during periods (it's easy to mistake endometriosis for IBS), if there is pain on intercourse or if you suspect infertility, then ask to be referred to a (preferably female) gynaecologist (especially if tests so far have revealed nothing).

Hints for Healthy Hormones

'Long term change requires looking honestly at our lives and realising that it's nice to be needed but not at the expense of our health, our happiness and our sanity.'

Ellen Stern
From *Meditations For Women Who Do Too Much*
by Anne Wilson Shaef

Now for the positive stuff! Having covered a few of the horrors associated with hormonal imbalances, let's see what else can be done to relieve these miserable conditions.

1 Most importantly – **See your GP for a check-up**. A priority should be to eliminate the possibility of other conditions with similar symptoms. For example, any unexpected and otherwise unexplainable pain, discharge or bleeding, especially between periods, should be investigated at once.

2 If you are taking – or are offered – **HRT** or the **PILL**, contact *What Doctors Don't Tell You* and obtain their reports on these two important subjects before you come to any final decisions about stopping or starting

medication. This is such an important point that I make no apologies for emphasizing it. Refer to the Directory or to Recommended Reading for details.

3 If you suffer from **hypoglycaemia**, deal with it. You are far less likely to see improvements unless you do this. The hints detailed here should help but check out Chapter 4 on Hypoglycaemia too. Some people who take diuretic drugs find that it makes hypoglycaemia symptoms worse. This does not apply, however, to naturally beneficial diuretic foods (see below).

4 Whatever your age, **avoid low-calorie diets** and forget about the battle to lose a pound or two. Women with a bit of comfortable padding who are properly nourished appear to be less at risk of hormonal disorders and brittle-bone disease than those who strive to be skinny. Remember the old saying: Better ten stone of curves than seven stone of nerves! During the menopause, specialist fat cells help to produce small quantities of oestrogen in order to reduce the risk of brittle bones occurring. So if you're a bit heavier because of the menopause, console yourself with the fact that Mother Nature really does know best.

5 Give up **salt**, salty snacks and processed, packaged foods which contain added salt. Change the way you flavour your food. Experiment with herbs and spices. Change to sea salt and then cut down very gradually over a period of several weeks. Low-sodium salt is another option but is not usually considered suitable for anyone with high blood pressure or those on diuretic drugs as it can disrupt the balance of potassium in the body.

6 Check **food labels**. Anything with the words sodium,

monosodium glutamate (MSG), sodium bicarbonate or
salt should be avoided or at least used less often.

7 Cutting down on **sugar**, sugary foods, artificial
   sweeteners and refined products made with white flour
   also helps.

8 Check for **food allergies**. I have found sensitivity to
   wheat and to cow's milk to be common amongst those
   with PMTS and menopausal symptoms. Intolerance to
   certain foods can also cause 'allergic oedema' which, to
   all intents and purposes, has the same symptoms as
   straightforward water retention. No one is really sure
   why allergies can cause this problem but it may be
   because the system is seeking to saturate the cells with
   fluid in an effort to 'wash away' irritating substances.
   Inflammation is also the body's natural response to
   invasion by unwanted imports. Whether this proves to be
   the case or not, my own experience with patients has
   been that removal of common allergens such as salt,
   refined corn or wheat cereals, bread, cow's milk, orange
   juice, corn, chocolate and sugar helps most towards
   reducing allergy-related imbalances and pre-menstrual
   bloating.

9 **Eat plenty of calcium-rich foods** such as sheep's or
   goat's yoghurt, buttermilk, canned salmon, canned
   sardines, curd cheese, dried figs, unblanched almonds,
   brazil nuts, oats, brown rice, pulses, seeds, tofu, fresh
   herbs, green and root vegetables. If these nourishing
   foods figure regularly in your diet, you should not lose
   anything by avoiding cow's milk. Be cautious, however,
   about taking separate calcium supplements without
   professional guidance.

10 Increase your intake of foods which are rich in **potassium** and **magnesium**; both help to keep sodium in balance. Good sources are fresh fruits, salad produce, vegetables, dried fruits, pulses, lean meat, fresh fish, soya, nuts (not peanuts), seeds, garlic, ginger and wholegrains. Grapes, raw carrots, raw beetroot seem especially helpful. Avoid pre-cooked beetroot – it usually contains preservative and is very unlikely to contain the same level of goodness as the raw, unadulterated beetroot.

11 Apples, cucumber, parsley, watermelon, watercress and dandelion leaves are not only nutritious but **naturally diuretic** too.

12 **Legumes** (pulses) and particularly **soya beans** are a healthy addition to any diet but may be especially important to those with hormonal imbalances. Although still a controversial area, researchers point to the fact that soy products (and some herbs and vegetables, including celery, fennel, parsley and linseeds) contain small amounts of natural substances called phytoestrogens which, although much weaker in activity than synthetic oestrogen, do not appear to have any unpleasant side effects. Studies show that Japanese women, who tend to eat larger amounts of these foods than Westerners, have far less incidence of hot flushes and other menopausal symptoms. Pulses are also very effective at helping to balance glucose levels in the blood and so are highly recommended to diabetics, hypoglycaemics – and those with pre-menstrual cravings.

13 **Don't boil** your vegetables in gallons of bubbling water; it reduces nourishment, particularly potassium and

Vitamin C. Steaming, stir-frying, casseroling and baking
are better for you. Or why not wok it?

14 Improve elimination of wastes. **Keep your colon
healthy**. Eat more dietary fibre.

15 Follow a **regular detox** as set out in my *Food Combining
2 Day Detox*.

16 **Drink more water**, between meals and first thing in the
morning too. But not directly from the tap. Filter it first.
There are several reasons for this caution. Fluoride and
chlorine in tap water do not seem to be helpful to any of
the conditions mentioned in this chapter. Now reports
suggest that excess fluoride may actually weaken the
bones and teeth. In addition, levels of the toxic metal,
lead, may be higher if you live in a soft-water area. Lead
can increase the risk of high blood pressure. But take
care to choose a filter that knocks out most of the nasties
but doesn't disturb the calcium levels too much (the pack
label should tell you).

♦ Surprising as it may sound, not drinking enough water
can *increase* fluid retention and aggravate other
symptoms such as irritable bowel syndrome and
constipation. Up your fluid intake and it can help
improve sodium/potassium ratios and flush trapped
fluid out of your system. But remember that water is
the key. You're most unlikely to achieve beneficial
results by downing gallons of tea and coffee. These
beverages can be beneficial in small amounts but
excesses could be counterproductive, making matters
much worse by overworking your kidneys. If you suffer
with breast tenderness or breast lumps or are at risk
from osteoporosis, I would advise removing caffeine

from the diet entirely since it seems to aggravate symptoms.

♦ If you don't have access to your filter (away from home, for example), then choose *non*-carbonated mineral water for emergency use. Drink the fizzy stuff for pleasure if you like it but don't rely on it as a daily water replacement. Why spend your whole life breathing out carbon dioxide and then gulp away at the bubbles in fizzy water? I keep small bottles of non-carbonated water handy and refill them from my filter unit for car journeys etc.

17 **Lighten up**. Don't let negative stress take over your life. Being habitually 'hyper' or in a state of constant anxiety is likely to increase production of the very hormones which cause your PMTS, enticing your cells to retain water and aggravate bloating.

18 Improving the digestion definitely seems to help those who suffer with PMTS, menopausal problems, fluid retention and bloating.

19 Extend yourself a little and **take a bit more exercise**. You know whether you are doing enough at the moment! Brisk walking, swimming, sensible workouts – anything aerobic is good. Lung capacity improves, bowel and kidneys function more efficiently; in fact, all routes of elimination are enhanced, helping you to get rid of unwanted garbage. Abdominal exercises are essential, helping to tone the pelvic contents, improve circulation and relieve congestion. So is sensible weight-lifting. Try two 1.35-kilo (3-pound) hand weights (dumbbells) that you can add to as strength and tone improves. Packs usually come with exercise diagrams. Regular physical

activity also helps to reduce stress and give you added protection against brittle bones!

20 *Don't cut down too far* on **quality protein** (yoghurt, eggs, fish, organic chicken, lean lamb, soya and other pulses, etc.) because you've heard that protein is bad for the kidneys and therefore might increase fluid retention. True, gross excesses of protein might do that but protein deficiency can do the same. Some experts believe that a high-protein, low-allergen diet and nutritional supplements are probably the safest and most effective way of maintaining or restoring hormonal balance. This has certainly been my own experience. Those who choose not to eat meat or fish can find valuable protein from vegetable sources, nuts, pulses, yoghurt, and so on. Beef, pork and factory-farmed poultry are best avoided even if you are not vegetarian. Organic poultry, lean lamb, game and fresh fish are good alternatives.

21 Check out the kinds of **fats and oils** you are using but *don't cut back too far*. Too little can be as dangerous as too much. Avoid fatty foods, fry-ups, cakes, pastries, pies, burgers and other food high in fat. Steer clear of anything which has 'hydrogenated vegetable oil' on the label – including processed margarine-type spreads. Use extra virgin olive oil for cooking and a little butter or non-hydrogenated margarine for spreading. If you buy polyunsaturates, choose only the cold-pressed kinds (the label will tell you) and keep for cold uses only – don't cook with them; not only is the nutritional value destroyed, researchers suspect a link between damaged oils and major illness such as heart disease and cancer.

♦ Time and time again, I have found that women with

the most severe PMTS and menopausal symptoms have followed low-fat diets for long periods of time. When the fatty nutrients are replaced, there is nearly always a significant improvement.

22 Make every effort to include **fresh oily fish** in your diet twice each week as well as almonds, Brazils, pumpkin seeds, sunflower seeds, avocado and top quality cold-pressed oils (buy the best you can afford).

♦ Health-food stores are the best places to find good quality cold-pressed oils and spreads although most supermarkets and grocery stores will stock extra virgin (first pressing) olive oil. (Avoid 'pure' olive oil; it isn't always the best.)

23 **Chiropractic**, **reflexology**, **acupuncture**, **herbalism** and **homoeopathy** have all demonstrated their value in relieving menstrual, pre-menstrual and menopausal symptoms, balancing the system and improving wellbeing. However, it can be difficult to decide which therapy is best for you. Fortunately, a number of health centres now offer consultations with qualified staff who can assess your needs and point you in the right direction. And talk with your GP; you may find some of these therapies available in your local surgery. In the case of aromatherapy and reflexology, there are many self-help measures that you can put into practice at home. *Aromatherapy – A Guide For Home Use* by Christine Westwood and *Aromatherapy – Simply For You* by Marion Del Gaudio Mak (£1.99 each – both from Amberwood Publishing) are an inexpensive place to begin. Also useful is *Reflexology – A Step By Step Guide* by Ann Gillanders.

TOP TIP Three useful essential oils to keep in your first-aid cabinet are *Geranium*, for its hormonal balancing properties; *Frankincense*, to comfort and rejuvenate; and *Lavender*, to soothe and relax. If your periods are a pain or you feel drained as a result of heavy bleeding, add three drops each of these oils to 30ml (2 table-spoons or 1 fluid ounce) of almond oil. Use the mixture to massage into the abdomen, lower back, feet, shoulders and between the breasts. Applying gentle but firm massaging pressure around and above the ankle bones and to the ball and arch of each foot can help to relieve period pain. Some companies make ready-mixed oils especially designed for pre-menstrual and period problems.

24 Provide **instant relief from hot flushes** by using an
    Evian spray or water-filled atomizer. Keep one in your
    bag or briefcase and spray your face and neck
    throughout the day. It brings refreshing relief and is good
    for the skin. Also valuable if you work in a hot, dry or air-
    conditioned atmosphere, in front of a vDU screen and
    when in aircraft.
25 Conversely, if you suffer with uncomfortable periods,
    mittelschmerz or the pain of endometriosis – the **heat**
    from hot-water bottles, heated comfort pads and warm
    baths can be very soothing.
26 If you feel 'tight', tense or anxious, remember that
    restrictive clothing such as Lycra leggings, tight teddies or
    bras, and cinched waists can wind you up even further.
    Go for looser garments and **be comfortable**.
27 Get outside. **Fresh air**, **daylight** and sensible amounts of

sunlight help to regulate and balance the hormonal system and reduce stress.

28 Don't feel guilty about taking a day or two away from work. Go with the natural rhythms of your life. If you feel a bit below par because it's your 'time of the month', respond to your body's needs and **rest up**. If you really truly cannot take time off, at least try to avoid taking work home; relax as much as possible and enjoy a few early nights.

29 Consider **hormone testing**. Your GP can carry out a full hormone profile (blood test) which should include FSH (follicle stimulating hormone), LH (lutenizing hormone), prolactin, progesterone and oestrogen. Back these results with FHPT (Female Hormone Panel Test) which uses saliva samples to test hormonal levels throughout the monthly cycle. The FHPT is recommended to anyone who has any of the conditions mentioned in this chapter and is especially valuable for those with pregnancy problems, infertility, early ovulation and oestrogen/progesterone imbalances.

30 An ever-increasing stack of serious research shows that the right kind of **supplements** can be especially helpful in relieving hormonal distress and associated problems such as pre-menstrual migraine, irritable bowel syndrome and mood changes. However, that doesn't mean it's wise or necessary to pop piles of pills every day. Nor will the same set of supplements work in the same way for every woman. It may be necessary to try several different approaches and tailor them to personal needs. In most cases, however, it seems that a well-structured programme of only a few supplements can give essential

support to a varied diet, providing optimum doses of all
the vital nutrients.

31 If you are unsure about choosing the right supplements, I
would urge you to seek the advice of a **qualified
nutritionist**. The cost of one consultation is likely to be
far less than the purchasing errors you might make
without advice.

32 I would also strongly advocate a nutrition consultation
with a practitioner who has a good track record in
treating **candidiasis**. I never cease to be amazed at the
number of times hormonally related disorders and
candida problems turn up together.

The Inside Story

∾

Candidiasis/thrush

You've seen what yeast does to beer or bread. Well, one of the main perpetrators of a gas-distended abdomen is overgrowth of a yeast organism called *Candida albicans*. Everybody 'has candida', since it is a natural inhabitant of the human lumen. In a healthy gut, this fungus is kept in check by friendly intestinal flora. Damage occurs only when the normal ecology of the bowel is disturbed, allowing the yeast to proliferate. Once changed from Dr Jekyll into Mr Hyde, the yeasty beasty can then 'attack' the healthy membrane between the digestive tract and the bloodstream (or cause further breaches in an already damaged gut wall). Toxic waste products seep into the general circulation, in their turn disrupting the healthy functioning of almost any part of the body.

Sounds nasty?

It is.

But don't despair if you're a sufferer. Even if you haven't found any so far, there really is lots of qualified, practical help around.

So read on.

In case you are confused by the terminology here's some help.

Candida albicans is the name of the yeast fungus itself. If you see the term *Monilia albicans* anywhere, that's just another label for the same fungus.

Thrush (sometimes also referred to as Candidosis) is the common name for the yeast infection caused by an overgrowth of *Candida albicans* – usually in the mouth, throat or genital areas.

Candidiasis is a term used by candida specialists to describe systemic yeast overgrowth – in other words, when it invades and affects the whole body.

The word 'candida' is often used interchangeably as an abbreviation for both the yeast and the condition it causes. Probably because it's easier to say.

Since systemic candidiasis is not generally recognized by orthodox medicine (except in advanced cancer), most medical dictionaries and the majority of doctors use the three names of Candidosis, Candidiasis and Thrush to mean the same thing – fungal infection at a superficial surface level.

Thrush is usually most people's first clash with *Candida albicans*, often as a result of antibiotics, sometimes prescribed for acne or an infection following a cold – but very often for cystitis (see page 204).

Although unpleasant and uncomfortable, at this 'surface' level, both the cystitis and the thrush should be relatively easy to treat naturally – with diet and immune-boosting nutrients – without resorting to repeat prescriptions of antibiotics. However, the common and constantly repeating cycle of cystitis—antibiotics—thrush—cystitis—antibiotics is likely to weaken the immune system and drive the yeast 'underground', especially if there are other underlying health problems (see boxes below).

Paradoxically, when *Candida albicans* has taken a firm grip on the gut, it may be the case for some people that thrush appears to clear up, only to return to the surface as the system is cleansed and healing takes place.

Some doctors find the suggestion of systemic candidiasis occurring in the general population hard to accept, particularly if there are no visible signs of yeast infestation. Whilst they agree upon the existence of vaginal and oral thrush (and on systemic candidiasis in patients suffering terminal illness), many remain resistant to the idea that this 'harmless' yeast could otherwise create such internal havoc.

It's not as if this is a new or simply fashionable condition. As long ago as 1931, doctors researching an illness with almost identical problems coined the phrase 'carbohydrate dyspepsia', to describe collective symptoms such as gas, bowel discomfort, irritable bladder, bloating, muscle pain and unexplained fatigue. Treatment involved the restriction of sweet

and starchy foods, and supplementation of pancre-
atic enzymes, probiotics and vitamins – not dissimi-
lar to today's recommendations.

In the late 1970s, Dr C. Orian Truss presented
research suggesting that a common mould, *Candida
albicans*, could be the trigger for an almost exactly
similar set of symptoms which he classified under
the general heading of Dysfunctional Gut Syndrome.

However, as far as orthodox science was concerned, the concept of a physical cause remained
unproven. Conventional medicine took the view
that most symptoms were 'probably psychiatric in
origin'. As this book goes to the publishers, important clinical studies into candidiasis are underway.
Evidence accumulated so far sees an 'all in the mind'
explanation as extremely unlikely!

Encouragingly, an increasing number of GPs are
already accepting the presence of candidiasis and are
willing to treat it. However, my own experience
with patients has been that, whilst the antifungal
drugs available on prescription can be effective in the
short-term, their benefits when used in isolation are
not prolonged. Far greater improvements seem to
accrue when anti-fungals are used with improved
diet and other lifestyle changes.

THE SYMPTOMS OF CANDIDIASIS

These are legion, making it easy to see why the condition
is so often missed – or misdiagnosed. The ones most
commonly presented are listed here:

Aching	Lethargy
Anxiety	Loss of libido
Bloating	Menstrual problems
Bowel problems	Muscle pain
Cravings	Nausea
Cystitis	Palpitations
Depression	Persistent infections
Digestive discomfort	Poor concentration
Dizziness	Poor coordination
Dry cough	Skin eruptions
Fatigue	'Spaced-out' sensations
Headaches or migraine	Stiff joints
Hypoglycaemia	Weight gain
Impaired recall	Vaginal dryness

Some of the most likely **causes** or **triggers** include: adrenal exhaustion; antibiotics; diets high in sugar; environmental and chemical overload; excess alcohol; HRT; low thyroid function; poor immunity; poor liver function; poor quality diet; protracted stress, and the contraceptive pill.

Of all these, at least from my own practice experience, **poor immunity** has to be the major factor in the explosion of candidiasis. According to leading Candida specialist, Sherridan Stock: 'A weak immune system appears to be the norm these days, the main reason for which, in our opinion, is nutrient deficiency. Almost every nutrient known has a role to play in creating immunity, and since most individuals exhibit multiple nutrient deficiencies, they inevitably have chronically impaired immune systems.'

I see the rise of candidiasis also depending very much on 'overload'. In other words, a properly nourished body may be well equipped to cope with short periods of stress, exhaustion, illness, chemical exposure, etc. Add frequent courses of antibiotics to a diet high in sugar and lacking in dietary fibre, drop in a few viruses and heavy doses of petrochemical fumes for good measure, pile on the stress and ignore the need for rest and sleep, and you are well on the way to breaking point. Every detrimental move makes it easier for *Candida albicans* to escalate and intensify.

THE ALL-IMPORTANT IC VALVE

Positioned just inside the right hip bone, near to the appendix, is the ileo-caecal valve (ICV). The main purpose of this one-way junction is to prevent the contents of the large intestine back-flowing into the small intestine. Not only do the symptoms of autointoxication which result from a faulty ileo-caecal valve bear a close resemblance to those of systemic candidiasis, it's likely that a defective ICV could exacerbate the candida condition and vice versa. Indeed, leading practitioners in the treatment of candidiasis believe that the two conditions of small bowel toxicity and overgrowth of *Candida albicans* often co-exist.

The term 'autointoxication' was first coined by Dr Ilya Metchnikoff in his book *The Prolongation of Life* (G.P. Putnam 1908) to describe what happens when

harmful toxins, produced by disease-promoting bacteria, are absorbed into the bloodstream.

It has nothing to do with being three sheets to the
wind or in any way the worse for drink.

HELP FOR CANDIDA SYMPTOMS

Help reduce candida symptoms by doing this simple
exercise every day:

Lie on the bed and make sure that you are comfortable.

Beginning just inside the right hip bone near the
crease of the leg, use the pads of the fingers to massage
the abdomen.

Work your way up towards the waist, across the belly
to the left-hand side and down again until you are level
with the left hip bone.

Then massage, left to right, across the middle of the
abdomen, and back again so that the whole of the area
is covered.

If you do not have strong fingers or suffer with arthri-
tis in your hands, massage will be easier if you lubricate
the fingers with a little olive oil. Or ask your partner to
carry out the massage for you.

Practised regularly, abdominal massage will help to
tone the muscles and strengthen the IC valve.

The presence of *Candida albicans* can also foster or
aggravate a number of other conditions including
migraine, hypoglycaemia, acne, eczema, psoriasis,
urticaria, hyperactivity, pre-menstrual syndrome,
asthma, food allergies, ear infections, hypothy-

roidism, irritable bowel syndrome and ME/Chronic
Fatigue Syndrome.

Successful treatment requires a several-pronged
'annihilate and nurture' programme. Kill off the
invasive yeast with anti-fungal supplements and
boost the immune system to protect against further
attack. The self-help measures provided in *Hotline to
Health* are those that patients tell me they have found
most effective.

However, I would strongly recommend that these
suggestions are used in conjunction with professional guidance. Candidiasis is a complex condition,
the treatment of which, I believe, requires the support of an experienced and qualified practitioner.

Above all, please don't launch into a restricted
dietary regime in the belief that, by avoiding long
lists of different foods, your candidiasis will give up
the ghost. There may be short-term relief but
drastic dietary measures are far more likely to lead
to worsening deficiencies and consequent mal-
nourishment. Poor immunity and lack of nutrients
are two of the most likely reasons why *Candida albicans* picked on you in the first place. So don't cut
calories. Eating healthily and well is essential to
full recovery. Apart from the suggestions mentioned here, leave the initial guidance on foods to
your nutritionist.

OVERLEAF ARE TWELVE IMPORTANT MOVES FOR YOU TO
MAKE WHILE YOU ARE WAITING TO SEE A
PRACTITIONER.

1 Get into the food-combining habit. A good place to start would be to follow my *Food Combining In 30 Days*. I'm thrilled to hear that it has helped so many candida sufferers. Details under Recommended Reading.

2 Drink more water – preferably filtered.

3 Drink cold-pressed aloe vera juice every day.

4 Cut all sugar, wheat and yeast from your diet.

5 For the time being, bypass any very ripe fruit. When you do eat fruit, enjoy it separately from other foods and you will digest it more efficiently.

6 Avoid all margarines and polyunsaturated cooking oils.

7 Use only extra virgin olive oil for salad dressings and for cooking. Use small amounts of butter for spreading.

8 Massage your abdomen (and ICV) with olive oil every day.

9 Add garlic to your cooking or, if you don't like the taste, take a garlic product. Candida hates garlic.

10 Avoid ordinary cow's milk completely and absolutely. Make sure that any you do buy is organic but keep that to a minimum, especially in the early stages of treatment. All supermarkets now stock organic milk.

11 Do eat plain bio-yoghurt daily. If possible, choose one made from sheep's or goat's milk but, if you can't find either of these, go for a quality live yoghurt made from organic cow's milk.

12 Buy two very important and extremely helpful books: *Beat Candida Through Diet* by Gill Jacobs (Vermilion) and a*The Practical Guide to Candida* by Jane McWhirter (Green Library), which contains a UK Directory of practitioners.

Irritable Bowel Syndrome

IBS is, essentially, a simple non-life-threatening disorder involving muscular spasm and inflammation in the large colon. Yet the agony and anguish it can cause are far from simple. A common condition and yet one associated with some extremely unpleasant symptoms and handicapped by a host of horror stories linked to misdiagnosis.

For example, a report in the *Scottish Medical Journal* tells the tale of a group of IBS patients who waited an average of seven years before a firm diagnosis of their condition was made. In an investigation carried out at the University of Edinburgh Gastrointestinal Unit, the case notes of six IBS sufferers were examined. Five of the six were referred for psychiatric assessment – although none was actually diagnosed with any psychiatric disorder. They each saw a minimum of six different specialists and yet many of the hospital doctors involved were not aware of the investigations already carried out elsewhere. Between them, these patients suffered a range of major operations, one person being sent for surgery seven times, another for six.

Discussions with other practitioners would suggest that this kind of scenario is not uncommon. Until quite recently, IBS was believed to be nothing more than a psychosomatic disorder.

Signs and symptoms

Confusingly for the patient, IBS has several

other names, including 'colicky bowel', 'nervous bowel', 'spastic colon', 'mucous colitis' and 'non-inflammatory bowel disease'.

INTERMITTENT OR DOMINANT IBS SYMPTOMS

These may include:

Abdominal pain

Anal soreness or irritation

Backache

Bleeding (rectal)

Bloating

Constipation

Diarrhoea

Flatulence

Headaches

Incomplete evacuation

Incontinence or leakage

Lethargy

Mucusy stools

Painful periods

Proctalgia fugax – intense rectal pain

Rapid breathing

Tiredness

Weight fluctuations

There seems little doubt that emotions have a direct effect upon motions since stress, anxiety, jaw clenching and bruxism (teeth grinding) and depression are also high on the list.

LIKELY CAUSES OR TRIGGERS OF IBS

Allergies or food intolerance, especially to lactose, milk
    protein, gluten, wheat or yeast
Being physically run down or feeling emotionally low
Bowel infection
Candida albicans
Chemotherapy or radiotherapy treatment
Disorders of the nervous system
Drug side effects
Gynaecological problems
Inadequate digestive enzymes
Intestinal parasites
Low levels of stomach acid
Nutrient deficiencies
Poor digestion
Poor quality diet
Relationship conflicts
Some types of iron supplements, such as ferrous
    sulphate
Surgery
Stress
Work pressure

IBS sometimes co-exists with pre-menstrual syndrome
and a disorder called fibromyalgia – painful and inflamed
tendons, muscles and ligaments and chronic fatigue.
Fibromyalgia has been described as 'having a whole-
body headache'. Symptoms may be worse during an IBS
attack or in the week before a period begins. Experts
have yet to determine the reasons for the link.

Getting on your nerves?

Although stress can be a significant factor, it doesn't mean that IBS is all in the imagination. Anxiety, nutrient deficiency or inherited neurological problems can 'irritate' the nerves which control bowel function. Like crossed wires at the telephone exchange, when the messages get mixed up, the bowel may empty more frequently – or less frequently than is considered normal.

On the psychological side, some IBS sufferers complain of being dominated by relationship conflicts (often with parents) where they may feel suffocated or trapped. Where constipation is dominant, there may be a reluctance to 'let go', to give anything away. Where diarrhoea has the upper hand, some people express fear and loneliness bound up with over-anxiety. And as appears to be the case in many bowel disorders, there may be stored anger and unexpressed feelings.

The medical solution

Peppermint-based antispasmodics (which are designed to help relax the muscles of the intestines) and anti-cholinergics (which control the contractions in the gut) are two of the most common prescriptions offered to IBS sufferers. Other options include laxatives to make you go and diarrhoea suppressants to do the opposite. None is recommended for continuous use.

A seemingly innocuous alternative which may be advocated is bran. But it doesn't suit everyone. If you've been advised to eat more of it, hang on.

Encouragingly, there are a number of gentle, yet effective approaches to the management of irritable bowel and other disorders of the colon. Try them and you may not need to resort to long-term medication.

CHECKLIST

Dietary and lifestyle hints for easing digestive and bowel disorders:

♦ A nutrient-dense, allergen-free diet and plenty of fluid are the cornerstones to the relief of many a grumpy gut. **Diet used in conjunction with other therapies** often has more value than if used alone. Conversely, relaxation and other techniques can be more effective if supported by a healthy diet. Stress management is vital.

♦ Learn to **relax**. Easier said than done? Consider yoga, learn TM (transcendental meditation), qi gong, autogenic training or t'ai chi. It really is worth going to local classes. Ask at your adult education centre or library for information.

♦ **Exercise your insides** with regular deep breathing exercises. Five minutes on waking and another five before settling down to sleep are usually enough to make the difference. Chinese philosophy has it that distress, anxiety and sadness lead to dysfunction of the large intestine by injuring the lungs. Improving the quality of breathing can increase energy flow between those organs. I have seen significant improvements in patients who have introduced simple daily deep-breathing exercises into their routine.

♦ The **traditional Chinese medicine** (TCM) approach using acupuncture and herbs has also been shown to be helpful,

especially for irritable bowel syndrome (IBS). In TCM, anger
and worry cause stagnation of energy in the liver and
spleen, resulting in gastrointestinal dysfunction.

◆ **Hypnosis** is worthy of consideration. A study carried out
at the University Hospital of South Manchester, England
(and reported in the *Lancet* in July 1992) found that
hypnosis had a calming effect on the gut, reduced pulse
rate and slowed the breathing. I have found that
reflexology, deep-breathing exercises and aromatherapy
have similarly beneficial effects. Some patients have
reported that their condition improves following sessions
of spiritual healing.

◆ **Daily physical activity** such as walking, swimming,
cycling, rebounding and skipping really do make a
difference. Simple stretching exercises done before and
after vigorous activity tone the muscles and reduce the risk
of spasm and cramp. I met someone quite recently who
admitted that the only time her bowels functioned
properly was during her annual walking holiday – when
she was exercising every day and feeling more relaxed.
Research shows that regular exercise coupled to a healthy
diet containing sufficient dietary fibre can lower the risk of
some bowel disorders by as much as 40 per cent.

◆ **Massage** the abdominal area daily with olive oil or olive oil
cream. Pay particular attention to your ileo-caecal valve.
This junction between the small and large intestines is
wont to suffer from poor muscle tone, allowing back flow
of poisonous wastes and a build-up of toxicity – just dandy
for an already irritable and sore system! The symptoms of
autointoxication which result from a faulty ileo-caecal valve
(headaches, lethargy, aching, dizziness, bloating, nausea

and other digestive disturbance) bear a close resemblance to those of *Candida albicans*. Apart from this important area, make sure you also massage the ascending colon, transverse colon and descending colon.

♦ **Food combining** can be an excellent way to improve digestion and absorption, a fact confirmed by former patients and by other practitioners. My own personally devised food-combining strategy has been developed over several years and is designed to be nutrient-dense and free from common allergens. It has also proved to be beneficial in improving the absorption of nourishment, speeding up transit time, relieving indigestion and constipation, and reducing bloating. If you suffer from Crohn's disease, candidiasis, ulcerative colitis, malabsorption, digestive discomfort, diverticulitis or IBS, it's worth giving food combining a try.

♦ Drink **aloe vera juice** every day. There is a great deal of research now available which demonstrates the soothing, healing capabilities of biogenic aloe vera juice in the treatment of digestive and bowel disorders. It seems particularly helpful for irritable bowel syndrome, ulcers, ulcerative colitis, Crohn's disease, hiatus hernia, acid reflux, nausea, candidiasis, indigestion and stomach upsets; comforting, too, after a heavy night out! Aloe also eases inflammation and may help promote healthy gut flora. If you suffer with piles, anal irritation, thrush or cystitis, diluted aloe makes a soothing douche.

To drink aloe vera juice, take 40ml (about 8 teaspoons) first thing in the morning, once or twice during the day – between meals – and again before bedtime. As a douche, dilute 20ml of aloe juice in 250ml water (otherwise translated as approximately 4 teaspoons in half a pint). Replace the bottle cap securely, keep your juice in the refrigerator and use it up within a month. A word of caution, however. Quality cold-pressed aloe juice can be hard to come by. Cheaper brands may not only be ineffective but can taste extremely bitter whereas a quality product makes a very pleasant, refreshing, cleansing and calming drink. Trust me. I made the same mistake.

♦ Don't get emotional about your motions but do try to understand a little about how your body works and respond to your gut's intelligence. If you receive a message that you need to visit the lavatory, **answer the call**. Don't wait until your bad-tempered bowel has gone back to sleep. It may not wake up again for days. However busy you are, don't be afraid to let your bowel rule your brain.

♦ Some practitioners recommend visiting the toilet 20 minutes after each meal (whether or not you feel the need to go) as this can help establish a **natural reflex** to open the bowels. If nothing else, it's one way of escaping for a period of quiet meditation! Just don't take the portable telephone with you! Return any calls when you're free or let them ring you again.

♦ **Don't strain**. Be patient. Just because we live in a world that demands instant mash, instant cash and instant coffee, don't push your body into performing instant defecation. If you follow the advice in this chapter, your bowels should open naturally when they are ready. Straining only increases the risk of piles and anal fissures, and weakens the muscles in the bowel wall.

♦ If regularity is a problem and motions tend to be sluggish,

practise some toilet training while you're watching the back of the door. Experts advise the following:

- ℘ Wait for the urge to empty and don't put it off once you feel the need to get up and go.
- ℘ Bear down only momentarily to allow the anal sphincter (the valve at the end of the back passage) to open.
- ℘ If necessary, help evacuation by deep slow breathing so that the abdomen moves in and out and the gut relaxes.
- ℘ Massaging the abdomen whilst sitting on the toilet not only encourages bowel emptying but improves muscle strength and tone.
- ℘ It can also help to raise the feet off the ground and rest them on two or three heavy books, a pile of magazines or an upturned washing-up bowl. This action places the body into a semi-squatting position and relaxes the colon.

♦ It is believed by many practitioners that an imbalance of intestinal bacteria (too many bad bugs in the gut) is often the starting point for disease. The levels of beneficial organisms that live there can be damaged in several different ways including surgery, anaesthetics, poor quality diet and, of course, antibiotics or any general drug treatment. **Restoring damaged flora** with supplements of *Lactobacillus acidophilus* and *Bifido bacterium* (sometimes called probiotics) has many benefits for those with bowel and digestive disorders; they include regulation of peristalsis (the contracting and relaxing action of the muscular wall), increased absorption of vital nutrients and reduction in inflammation and flatulence. Probiotics improve the consistency of bowel motions and reduce both diarrhoea and constipation. They reduce the attachment of pathogenic organisms to the gut wall; in other words, discouraging the bad guys from taking up residence.

If you are taking a course of **acidophilus**, a good time to swallow it is with your linseeds and water first thing in the morning. It has more chance of being effective if it slides through the system with the linseeds than if allowed to shoot down with water only.

Unfortunately, independent tests have shown that some **probiotics** just don't make the grade and can be not only a waste of money but potentially hazardous. I have found those produced by Blackmores and Biocare to be the most effective. A six-month course is recommended to anyone with bowel or digestive malfunction and should be considered essential after antibiotics. Once again, these supplements appear to have far greater impact when used in conjunction with an improved diet and other nutritional support.

TIP

If you are using grapefruit-seed extract in the treatment of candidiasis, Salmonella infection or gut parasites, always follow with a course of probiotics to help re-populate the tubes with healthy bacteria. Don't take the probiotics at the same time as the grapefruit seed.

◆ Daily helpings of **plain, live, bio-yoghurt** are gentle on the digestive system. Although the levels of friendly bacteria won't be as concentrated as in probiotic supplements, some should find their way through the stomach to the small intestine. Yoghurt made from sheep's or goat's milk is preferred. It's also worth knowing that, for most people, even cow's milk yoghurt is far easier to digest than straight cow's milk and provides a worthwhile source of well-absorbed calcium. Where reflux or acidosis is a problem, a spoonful of yoghurt can provide a side-effect-free alternative to antacid medications.

♦ To help calm an irritable bowel or an overactive nervous system, try **regular daily supplements** of multivitamins (make sure they contain all the main B vitamins as well as magnesium). Additionally, take separate capsules of either a quality Evening Primrose oil brand (for example, Efamol) or a GLA complex such as Pharma Nord Bio-Glandin or Biocare Mega GLA. Since multiple nutrient deficiencies, poor immunity and stress appear to be common to so many bowel and digestive disorders, this basic programme could offer valuable preventive medicine. Such a supplement may also be of value where there is family history of any kind of gut disorder. (For adults with sensitive digestions, two children's multivitamins or children's B-complex capsules are often better absorbed than one large adult dose.)

♦ **Vitamin C** is a vital nutrient in the easing of bowel disorders. Treat with caution any comments about 'extra Vitamin C only makes expensive urine' or 'Vitamin C causes diarrhoea'. Whilst it's true that excess amounts of this nutrient will spill over into the bladder and the bowel, it seems likely that such action is extremely beneficial. For example, regular daily supplements of Vitamin C can not only help guard against attacks of cystitis and reduce the risk of gastrointestinal infections but also, studies confirm, protect against ulceration and inflammation. C can also prevent the formation of cancer-initiating substances called nitrosamines, thereby reducing the risk of colon cancer and stomach cancer.

Check food labels and avoid anything which contains **nitrites** (such as sodium nitrite preservative). Nitrites can link themselves to proteins inside the body to form the carcinogenic nitrosamines mentioned above.

Anyone with troublesome bowel or digestive symptoms is strongly advised to take 1 or 2 grams of **buffered Vitamin C complex** every day. Patients with ulcerative colitis, diverticulitis or constipation should take 2 to 3 grams daily. The quality of the Vitamin C you choose is vitally important. The more gentle, buffered Vitamin C labelled magnesium ascorbate or calcium ascorbate seems to offer particular benefits over the cheaper plain ascorbic acid which has been known to cause indigestion and diarrhoea in some people.

♦ Supplements containing **herbal liquorice** can help to reduce inflammation and encourage healing of gastric ulcers. Useful too for heartburn, ulcerative colitis and Crohn's disease. In at least one clinical trial, a special form of liquorice was as effective as anti-ulcer medication. Liquorice also has mild laxative properties. Although not proven, there has been some suggestion that excesses of liquorice might increase fluid retention and disturb potassium levels in the body. However, this side effect does not appear to apply to low doses, and should not affect anyone who has a diet high in potassium-rich fresh

vegetables, salads and fruit. Ask your health store for
advice.

> An additional precaution: don't use liquorice if you have
> hypertension or are using diuretics or digoxin (digitalis).

♦ The herbal remedy **Slippery Elm** (in capsules or powder) is
soothing for all the mucous membranes that line the
digestive tract, calming inflammation and irritation
throughout the body. Especially helpful in cases of
indigestion, reflux, acidity, ulcers, IBS, ulcerative colitis,
diarrhoea, catarrhal conditions and cystitis. An essential
remedy for the first-aid cupboard. Some powders may be
sold in a wheat flour or lactose base so please check labels
for pure products in case wheat or milk are problem foods
for you.

♦ If **aluminium** is present in food, it can cause gas and
distension. For this reason, it is best to avoid aluminium
cookware. Check packet labels too – many dried foods
contain aluminium as an anti-caking agent.

♦ Be wary of proprietary indigestion remedies. Many of them
contain aluminium, too. An excellent alternative for
emergency use is **herbal Meadowsweet** (sometimes
combined with activated charcoal), available in tablets
from health-food stores. Activated charcoal not only
absorbs gas but also helps to bind and eject toxins from
the system. Meadowsweet has soothing antacid
properties, relieves distension and wind, helps combat
infection and is one of the best remedies for heartburn,
gastritis and the soreness of hiatus hernia.

♦ Use only soft, unbleached **toilet tissue** and wet wipes.
Keep the rectal area scrupulously clean (be particularly
vigilant if anal fissures or parasites have been a problem)

but do not use ordinary soap which strips the skin of its natural oils and can lead to further soreness and irritation.

♦ See a chiropractor or osteopath regularly. **Spinal manipulation**, especially of the thoracic and lumbar spine, can be very helpful in the treatment of all kinds of bowel and digestive malfunction, and candidiasis. Imbalances, particularly of the lumbar spine, may disturb normal blood flow and nerve transmission to the pelvis and abdominal organs.

♦ **Avoid** tight-fitting clothing, over-enthusiastic elastic and constricting belts.

Important note

If none of these things improves your condition, see a naturopath or doctor who is familiar with nutritional treatment and able to test for allergies and to isolate any underlying digestive disorders. Contact them and find out if they are willing to get together for a ten-minute 'meet and chat' before you commit yourself to a full appointment. (If travelling distances make this difficult, at least ask to speak personally with them on the telephone.) If they are too busy for you before treatment, they are unlikely to be there for you during or after!

Coping with Allergies

꒰

Allergy or Intolerance? Clearing up Confusion

Understanding your symptoms is an important part of successful treatment too. So, first of all, let's look at the difference between 'allergy' and 'intolerance', terms that are bandied around all over the place and are often misunderstood.

Put *very* simply and generally, allergies involve the immune system, and intolerances are linked to the digestion. But there's a bit more to it than that.

One of the main reasons for the confusion may be that quite a few of the symptoms of allergy also turn up in those who suffer with food intolerance.

What is an allergy?
The word 'allergy' means *altered reaction*, an abnormal response to a normal substance; the 'allergen' is usually something that occurs in everyday surroundings but which the body considers to be a foreign 'invader'.

Particles of one sort or another come into contact

with the body via the skin, lungs and digestive system all the time. A healthy system with a strong immunity will deal with these potential invaders so quietly and efficiently that you probably won't even notice, in other words, there were no particularly troublesome symptoms. When the immunity is weakened or the onslaught increases to unacceptable, uncontrollable levels, then we talk in terms of 'allergic reactions'.

It's possible to react violently to an allergen via the breathing apparatus (for example, a reaction to pollen or pet fur) as well as through the digestive system (for example, to peanuts or seafood). In susceptible people, the body sees these normally harmless substances as trespassing aliens and reacts accordingly. An unfortunate case of mistaken identity.

Here's what happens. (Skip this next paragraph if you're put off by long words which you don't need to remember anyway, but stick with it if you're interested. I'll try to make it speedy.)

When an allergen enters the body, the immune system calls up defence-force antibodies called Immunoglobulin E (IgE is easier to say). These, in turn, trigger the release of chemical messengers, including histamine, from white blood cells known as basophils and mast cells. Basophils circulate in the bloodstream and mast cells are found in the connective tissue of the skin, nose, lungs and digestive tract. Antihistamines are drugs prescribed to damp down the histamine reaction.

Taking Action Against Asthma and Allergies

TREATMENT TIPS

♦ Give your adrenals a rest and learn to relax. Managing stress is an important part of managing asthma and allergies. An over-stressed system is likely to create more cortisol and adrenalin than are needed. When produced in excess, these hormones suppress immunity and increase the risk of adverse reactions.

♦ Practise t'ai chi, meditation or other relaxation techniques. Consider regular reflexology treatment and/or aromatherapy massage as essential. Anyone interested in using massage at home is encouraged to read *Massage: A Step-by-Step Guide* by Yvonne Worth, *The Complete Book of Massage* by Clare Maxwell-Hudson or *A Complete Guide to Massage* by Susan Mumford. Massage of the back, chest and abdomen is known to help the breathing; gentle flowing movements are de-stressing and relaxing. However, anyone who suffers with (or is caring for someone who has) chronic asthma should consult a professionally qualified practitioner/teacher or attend recognized classes. Massage carried out incorrectly might make symptoms worse in extreme cases.

♦ Strengthen your resistance to attack by improving your lung function. Practise yoga and abdominal breathing exercises. Take singing lessons. Blow up balloons. Youngsters can blow through straws into a beaker of water or use bubble-blowing kits. Adults are also welcome to try this, of course, but perhaps not in a public place!

TRY THIS EXERCISE

Stand near an open door or window with hands behind your head and elbows pointing forwards. As you breathe in, move the elbows sideways, opening up the chest. When breathing out, move elbows so that they are pointing forwards again. A particularly helpful exercise for those who work in front of VDU screens. Keyboard work encourages a slouched posture and cramps the chest.

- Swimming (breast stroke), gentle rebounding, slow cycling (using an indoor machine) and walking are also recommended. Choose what appeals most to you – there is no need to do them all! The trick is to enjoy, go gently and not overexert yourself.
- See a McTimoney chiropractor for a course of treatment. Spinal misalignment appears to aggravate allergies and lung function. This very gentle form of chiropractic can be of real benefit. Regular check-ups reduce reactions and seem especially helpful to asthmatics.
- Find an experienced and qualified clinical ecologist or allergist who has a proven track record in treating allergic conditions and can carry out a range of recognized tests. If possible, try to arrange to be referred by your GP.
- Don't go into the garden (and keep windows closed) if anyone is cutting grass, ground clearing or pruning. And whilst we are all mindful of the connection between allergies and grasses, it's also worth remembering that huge quantities of pollen can drift from shrubs such as viburnum and buddleia and from conifers if they are disturbed by wind or gardening activity.

Be Diet-wise

Deciding which foods (if any) are the real trouble-makers can be a thorny problem. It is possible to have specific allergies to absolutely anything but equally important to realize that what causes a reaction in one person may not do so in another even if both suffer from allergies. A classic case of one person's meat being another person's allergen.

Mould can make matters worse

Foods which readily attract mould should be viewed with caution (even if you are not allergic to the foods themselves) since moulds are well-known allergy triggers. So make sure that you use only the freshest items. I always remember the advice given at a health lecture by nutrition expert Geoffrey Cannon that we should *eat food that goes bad before it goes bad!* (Think about it!) How wise. It is generally the case that the most nourishing foods are those that will, under normal circumstances, deteriorate the quickest: that is, fresh, whole, unadulterated produce. Processed and preserved foods that store for weeks or months are not likely to contain the same level of nourishment as their fresh equivalents.

Go easy!

So many different foods are potential triggers that you may think it's best to give up almost everything and exist on a very restricted diet.

Absolutely not.

Short-term exclusion diets can be helpful in some cases but it is *not necessary or safe* to follow them for long periods of time. Indeed, a few over-zealous allergy therapists have been criticized – probably with justification – for removing too many potential allergens from patients' diet for too long and not properly monitoring nutritional status and progress of symptoms. I cannot stress too strongly the need for vigilance when dealing with food allergies or intolerances.

Watch out for well-known troublemakers

This is the very short list of foods which I recommend are avoided – or at least reduced considerably – by anyone who is trying to improve their general health, whether they have allergies or not: Cow's milk, wheat-based cereals, 'squashy' mass-produced bread, sugar, and yeast and yeasty foods (stock cubes, yeast extracts, beer, etc.). These are items which have turned up repeatedly as problem foods, aggravating bowel and digestive disorders, bloating, candida, tiredness, weight problems and a range of other symptoms. There will always be those who don't go along with this view but I stick to my guns. If you are worried that you might be missing out on nutrients, don't – because you won't.

FAVOURITE FOODS

It's worth noting that patients often say they feel better when they concentrate on eating only their 'favourite' foods. Ironically, however, foods that figure prominently in the diet, that is, are eaten every day or several times a day, are often found to be the culprits. It makes working out what to eat and what to give up an extremely difficult task. If you give up favourites or cut back on them and feel worse for a while, that may indicate withdrawal symptoms. This scenario can also apply to migraine sufferers. The complicated nature of trying to sort out food allergies and intolerances makes practitioner support absolutely vital.

SUPPLEMENTS

♦ One of the treatments that I have found to be most effective in reducing allergic reactions is a course of **liver-cleansing herbs** such as **Silymarin** (milk thistle) or a combination of **dandelion** and **burdock**. There are a number of excellent products on the market, including Blackmores Herbal Springclean, Biocare HEPaguard 194 or their Silymarin Complex, Milk Thistle Vegicaps from Solgar and FSC Milk Thistle tincture; each as valuable as the other in stimulating, tonifying and detoxing the liver and digestive system. Choose one only (you don't need to take them all) and follow a three-month course. If you're a hayfever sufferer, begin early in the year, before the sneezing season starts.

♦ I have found that liver-cleansing herbs work well with Biocare's Histazyme, a nutrient complex that appears to reduce adverse reactions to a range of allergens.

♦ At the end of the three-month period, stop your herbs and change to a top quality **multivitamin/mineral complex** such as Solgar's VM 2000 and one or two grams of either FSC, Biocare or Blackmores **Vitamin C**. If funds allow, continue for nine months, returning to a three-month herbal programme at the beginning of next year. This combination has proved helpful in the treatment of hay fever, food intolerances and in reducing the frequency of colds.

> **Be aware** that the drugs used to treat allergies and asthma may reduce the levels of some nutrients in the system, including Vitamin B6, Vitamin C and magnesium. Ironically, low levels of these nutrients have been associated with a number of chronic airway diseases. Those who need regular medication for their asthma or allergy may see a reduction in side effects if they take a multivitamin/mineral capsule each day with a meal.

♦ **Vitamin C** is an essential nutrient for anyone with allergies since one of its chief characteristics is to inhibit the rise of histamine. Another is its ability to strengthen resistance to infection. Vitamin C has also turned up trumps in several studies with asthmatics, helping to improve lung function and enhancing resistance to airborne and environmental allergens such as cigarette smoke, traffic pollution and chemicals.

> **Note:** Whilst most multi complexes usually contain small amounts of Vitamin C, I have seen the best improvements with additional daily amounts; one or two grams (1000–2000mg) for adults and 500mg for children.

- **Bioflavonoids** can help to relieve sneezes, wheezes, coughing, sore eyes, irritation and itches. Like their common partner Vitamin C, flavonoids have a natural 'anti-histamine' action, inhibiting histamine release, reducing inflammation and strengthening capillaries. Beneficial sources of flavonoids are blackcurrant, bilberry, quercitin, rutin, hesperidin and ginkgo biloba. Those who are intolerant of citrus fruits should avoid brands of Vitamin C which contain citrus bioflavonoids.

- **For children** under 14 years, your health store should be able to supply a children's multivitamin/mineral complex that contains B vitamins, including B5, B6 and B12, magnesium, zinc, manganese and selenium plus extra Vitamin C as above. **Teenagers** over 14 years should be able to swallow the adult capsule.

- For all kinds of respiratory allergies but especially for hay fever, the herb **Echinacea** can be helpful in increasing resistance and reducing severity. I have had particular personal success using a combination of Echinaforce and Pollinosan tinctures (both by Bioforce) plus Blackmores Bio-C Vitamin C.

- **Vitamin B12** appears to be of benefit in both asthma and allergies. I have known some GPs who are willing to give a course of these inexpensive injections on prescription. Failing that, a three-month course of tablets, capsules or drops once a year seems to be just as effective. Try Biocare or Solgar brands.

  Note: Doctors may refuse to consider B12 on the basis that levels of B12 appear normal following a blood test. Whilst blood is an excellent medium for testing iron stores, it is not accurate for B12. Normal blood levels *do* *not* always indicate absence of deficiency. In therapeutic trials, subjects benefited even where there were no signs of clinical deficiency.

♦ A combination of **herbal and homoeopathic treatment** can bring about significant improvements although I have found they exert greater benefit if used in conjunction with diet and improvements to digestion and elimination. For children who use nebulizers, homoeopathic solutions may offer an alternative to drugs. Do consult a qualified homoeopath and involve your GP if possible.

♦ Two kinds of **essential fatty acids** (called Omega 3 and Omega 6) have been shown to be helpful in a wide range of different conditions. Fish oil and linseed oil belong to the Omega 3 group. Evening Primrose oil and other sources of GLA (gamma linolenic acid) such as borage oil come under the Omega 6 heading. It's wise to use one kind of oil from each category.

In the case of **Omega 6**, similar benefit would be gained in many conditions from using either Evening Primrose oil or an equivalent GLA product made from, say, borage oil, since both are good sources. In the specific cases of asthma and allergies (including hay fever), however, I have found Evening Primrose oil to be the most effective source – especially when treating children. The quality is important so buy the best EPO that you can afford, such as Efamol. Avoid cheaper 'one-a-day' brands and any which contain additives. Evening Primrose oil and Vitamin E are the only vital ingredients necessary in Evening Primrose oil capsules.

When it comes to **fish oil**, I have found the products known as Efamast and MaxEPA (available from pharmacies), Pharma Nord Bio-Marine, FSC Fish Oil 1000mg and Biocare's Mega EPA 1000mg to be of equal benefit; all are rich sources of the active ingredients EPA (eicosapentaenoic acid) and DHA (docosahexaenoic acid). Some patients may find fish oil and Evening Primrose oil available on prescription. It's worth asking the doctor.

Vegetarians, vegans or those with fish allergies should try the **linseed oil equivalent** (Biocare or FSC Organic Linseed 1000mg). But do use capsules, not bottled oil which has a very short shelf life and goes rancid extremely quickly. And take care not to confuse nutritional linseed oil with the kind used to treat wood!

For younger children capsules can be broken open and the contents mixed with food. Evening Primrose capsules can be pierced and the oil massaged into the child's abdomen or inside thighs daily (two good sites for absorption). This can be particularly helpful in cases of infant eczema and with young children who have asthma.

The importance of probiotics

Improving the level of friendly gut flora can help adults (and children) with allergies, asthma and eczema. Work carried out at Addenbrookes Hospital, Cambridge, England has established a connection between disturbed gut flora, food intolerances and irritable bowel syndrome.

SPECIAL OFFER

Pan Books publishes three of Kathryn Marsden's top-selling health titles:

All Day Energy Diet	£4.99
Food Combining 2 Day Detox	£4.99
Hotline to Health	£5.99

ZEST readers can order these books by credit card WITH FREE POSTAGE AND PACKING by phoning 01624 675137. All three books can be purchased together at the special price of £15 ALSO WITH FREE POSTAGE AND PACKING. You can also order by post by sending a cheque to Books By Post, PO Box 29, Douglas, Isle of Man IM99 1BQ.